All About Me Fitness!

{ **WRITTEN BY** *Denise L. Jackson* }

ISBN- 13:978-1467929622
ISBN-10:146792962X

Cover Design by Carrie Rockett

Printed in the United States of America

{DEDICATION}

I dedicate this book to every:

Senior Citizen;
keep telling us those stories, we love them

Morbidly Obese;
never feel less than, ever

Sedentary;
we are going to move, regardless how we feel

Office Workers/Home Base Entrepreneurs;
keep working but play also

Chronic pain sufferers and other health issues;
talk to God, He always listening

Uninspired/lazy people;
it could be worst, look at the line above

And of course, Darnell, my heart!

{ACKNOWLEDGEMENT/CONTRIBUTORS}

I would like to acknowledge all the contributors to this book and for the many experts I have spoken to on fitness and health for this underserved market. Your input has been invaluable.

Sally Shields www.sjcion.skinnyfiber.com

Diana McCalla www.cocoa101.com

Joni Lang www.oilessentials.com

Andy Lapointe www.traversebayfarms.com

Barbara Fanelli www.freekehlicious.com

Ruthie Smith www.ultimateliving.com

Annemarie McDermott www.crazyfornutrition.com

Dr. Joseph Artiss/ Dr. Catherine Jen www.mirafit.com

Barbara Turner www.energynaturalway.com

Dr. Randy Gilchrist www.theweightlossmindset.com

Heather Wolf www.jugglefit.com

Phil Black www.fitdeck.com

Ellen Miller www.isobreathing.com

Emilie Yount www.Fitandfabliving.com

Howie Shareff www.youcallthisyoga.org

Adrian Ramirez www.adrianspowerpilates.com

Ruth Smith www.sagewellnessla.com

Doug Sheppard www.janddfitness.com

Khadi Madama www.about.me/madamaconsulting

Rhonda H. Greene www.bodyinbalance757.com

Eduardo Barrera www.gravitywerks.com

Tom Rutlin www.walkingpoles.com

{TABLE OF CONTENTS}

{INTRODUCTION}

Before I go any further, this book is not just a book on how to lose weight. It is a book on how to get fit and healthy using different techniques along with different experts. Fit and healthy means you are taking steps in your life to maintain a certain weight, to create ideal numbers for blood pressure, cholesterol and a host of other things.

I used to like exercising when I was in my 20's. I don't like exercising now. I rather come home after being out all day, cook dinner, read, go on the Internet or watch TV. I rather get a root canal than to walk on a treadmill. I rather go into labor than do one of my BeachBody workout tapes. I know, I know, I am lazy when it comes to exercising. Yes, I am woman enough to admit it. But I also know that if I want to see my son get married, play with my grandchildren, travel well into my 80's, continue gardening, then I have to change my health and fitness routine.

I have so many DVDs and books on weight loss that they are all looking the same. Some may have a twist here and there but the bottom line is you have to do some serious movements and serious changes to how you utilize food to see results.

Since I had all of these books and DVDs I started looking at them and studying them and I was going back and forth with information and it was getting on my nerves. First of all most of the exercises shown were way too advanced for me. I could take some movements from one plan and add it to another plan but I had to delete some steps yet I could add some steps and this became way too confusing.

So I decided to go to my local bookstore and see what types of health and wellness books I could find for a person who is sedentary, works in an office, has a home based business and has three fibroids all in one book. Yeah, right.

Needless to say the bookstore was not much help to me. Sure, they had books, tons of them in this billion dollar industry, but nothing for me specifically.

Needless to say the bookstore was not much help to me. Sure, they had books, tons of them in this billion dollar industry, but nothing for me specifically.

I Google books for my criteria, exercises for a person who sits pretty much all day, sedentary, have fibroids tumors. They had plenty of fitness books but not anything all together. Was there a fitness and health program available for someone like me? Then I started thinking about others? What about senior citizens, what about people with chronic pain or other health problems? Is there any place where we could customize our fitness needs? Can we find a program that exercises the upper body because the lower body may be weak or what can be done in between working at a desk, waiting for a phone call at a call center or just watching TV? Are there tools, supplements and services that can help me with building my body and giving me the energy to be a productive person?

After not finding what I wanted I just put a simple question on the Internet? Does anyone have any lazy exercises that I can do?

The next day I could not believe the response. There

are literally hundreds of people out there who have the knowledge to create a fitness program just for you or who have products and tools to help with our fitness goals! For example, you may take some pills with certain food or drink and feel bad afterwards but I can do the same thing yet I feel perfectly fine. My point is this, we are all different. We are all in different stages of our lives when it comes to getting fit and healthy. We have to do things our way and not like everyone else. Shouldn't we have a choice on which type of exercise we should be doing? Shouldn't we have a choice on which supplements we would like to use for added nutrition and strength?

I decided to do a little research. Who are the people creating exercises and nutrition for people who may not be able to run a marathon or can't walk on a treadmill? Is there even a market for customize health and fitness plans? Are people asking for these types of plans? To tell you the truth I don't think people are asking or even demanding programs because we see what is advertise on TV and we see the programs are not for us and we just assume only a certain type of person should be fit and healthy. Not people like myself because if it was so, we could see programs being advertised on the TV. Before you know it we are going along in life not moving like we should be and we assume just because we don't see it then it just doesn't exist. This simply is not true. After getting the information I needed for my plan I decided why not have this information readily available to all who wants a custom fitness plan.

After talking to some of the fitness experts and business owners who market live foods, supplements and vitamins I decided to let them explain their products and how they could help others.

The book has chapters of fitness experts telling you how or what you can do to get fit and healthy. Do you know we have a former Navy Seal who created decks of cards for any type of fitness you can think of? We also have another company that has Green Miracle, a live food that helps you when you are having chemo or if you want a live, healthy food consistently in your diet. Since you have a variety to choose from why not questioned as many as you can and see if you could incorporate a little of each to make the perfect plan for you. You are bound to find the right fit for you. This book will ultimately be your go to guide to see what the latest tool to use is or the latest moves when it comes to your exercise plan.

Why should fitness experts and others assume just because they have a product it fits all of our needs? Those days are over!

Now are there more experts out there? Yes, of course there is. But for now we have a starting point with this book. As time goes on and we start questioning the billion dollars health and wealth industry and demanding custom programs we should begin to see positive changes.

I now know people should not have to skip exercising because they feel the programs marketing on TV are not for them. Why should fitness experts and others assume just because they have a product it fits all of our needs? Those days are over! For the health and wellness industry you need to start studying and creating programs and supplements for the underserved market. Study the body of a person who has fibromyalgia and create programs for that person. If a person is morbidly obese don't assume they are destined to stay that way. Help them and create programs and tools to make their fitness goal a success as well.

I now have choices and so do you! I will say this. I do not favor any fitness product, practices, supplements, fitness expert or any business over another located in this book. I think that would be unfair to you all when making your decision. You have to decide for yourself. One thing I did ask, the products had to be natural and not interfere with any medicines. I would suggest you check with your doctor before starting any exercise plans or taking any supplements. You decide that you are ready and not anyone else! If you want to contact a particular expert, by all means go ahead. They are there to serve you!

{ *I now have choices and so do you!* }

CHAPTER ONE

WEIGHT FOR ME

Growing up I was a slim girl. I could eat a Suzy Q cake and down it with a Pepsi and I was good for the next 5 hours. My stomach was flat as a pancake and weight was never an issue. My freshman year in college I was exactly 99 pounds. I will never forget because my doctor was filling out the form for my physical which the school had sent to me and he notice the address was in North Carolina and at the time I was living in Queens, NY. He said, "Why are you going so far away to school, there are great schools right here? Are you sure all 99 pounds of you are ready to leave mommy and daddy"? I answered, "Yes, all 99 pounds are ready to leave mommy and daddy".

Needless to say after college and the many years after that I did gain weight but was pretty okay with how I looked. After all I am 5 feet 8 inches so more added weight on my body didn't have me at the overweight stage yet. Now the day I went into labor I was 186 pounds but I felt that extra weight was warranted. After all I was eating for two. Soon after I gave birth my weight went back to normal and everything was lovely or so I thought.

A couple of years later working on Wall Street I would hang out after work for drinks and wings or whatever my colleagues wanted to eat and I notice my size 9-10's were fitting snug and I was beginning to get a gut. I literally panic. This can't be happening to me! I have to lose this stomach. I have to get back into my suits. I have given Casual Corner way too much money not to fit back in my clothes. I got the Jane Fonda tape and every day after work I would go into the basement while my son was playing with his cars and trucks and play Jane Fonda's exercise video in the VCR. Jane and I were best friends for at least 3 months straight. I was able to get back into my clothes and my stomach was looking like I wanted it to look, flat! After I lost approximately 20 to 25 pounds a few people told me to stop. I didn't need to lose any more weight.

As time moved on I left NY to pursue other dreams and passions and I settled in North Carolina. Moving to the south did take some getting used to because I was so accustomed to taking public transportation in NY. I found myself running for the bus or running for the train or going up

I literally panic. This can't be happening to me! I have to lose this stomach.

and down the stairs to catch a train or bus. I was constantly moving in NY. Here in North Carolina I was not. I would get in the car and drive to the store, work, home improvement store, doctor's office, etc and I was perfectly fine with that.

Then I decided to make a huge change in my life. I gave up smoking. One of the hardest things I have ever had to do. I failed several times so I decided to give this huge burden (well it was huge to me) to God and let Him deal with it. I guess He was urging me to try the Patch and within one week my desire to smoke or use the Patch was over. I have not picked up a cigarette since.

But don't congratulate me just yet. Yes, I have heard people sometimes pick up weight when they stop smoking, but OH

MY GOSH, 52 pounds! Yes, I did not make a typing error, 52 pounds. Throughout the years the weight was steadily creeping up and now instead of getting the Jane Fonda tape (yes, I still have it) I tell myself at least you are not smoking. It is as if I am going to hold on to the fact I quick smoking so now if I fail at anything else I can constantly use that lame, old tired excuse to make myself feel better. Well I needed to get over that because I've stopped smoking years ago. I also tell myself that I am going to

Needless to say I've found a fitness plan that works just for me. I've found some supplements that work just for me. You will find a plan that will work just for you as well.

start something on Monday, no matter what it is. Why do I do that? How much sense does that make if it is a Wednesday and I need to start changing some of my habits, why wait until Monday, what's wrong with Thursday or even Friday? This was my mentality for a long time, in fact for years.

So now we are in present day maybe 3 and half months ago and I have come to a realization. I am lazy when it comes to exercising or getting fit. I can clean my home, work in my garden or shop until I drop but I just don't feel like doing an exercise DVD or walk on a treadmill or use any other type of exercise equipment. Hey, at least I am honest. But I am also a realist. I know that being overweight is not healthy.

I also know that I have to change but I need to change my way. I wish I could be like some of the authors who are telling us how disciplined they were in changing their habits and lifestyles and what they did to become this size

4. But I represent a lot of people out there that are not disciplined nor easily swayed to change just because you've changed and now you are fit as a fiddle. Now, don't get me wrong. My heart wants to change. I have several dieting books; I have an elliptical in my bedroom and a treadmill in my garage. I have seen so many shows about people losing the weight. Do you know, to be honest, watching those people lose weight is wonderful and God bless them all but it never did nothing for me. The shows never motivated me one iota. But we will talk about motivation later. One thing for sure, some of us can look at people all day long lose weight but if we are not ready to lose the weight or get fit, nothing is going to motivate you to do so.

So, what was my plan? How was I going to conquer the battle of the weight when I knew I like looking at TV or going on the computer, working on my business or reading a book? How was I going to get fit and healthy, knowing I was lazy, sedentary and had fibroid tumors? Yes, some of us are just plain lazy. When you can admit it, trust me, a load is lifted off your chest. You no longer have to feel guilty of not walking around the school track which is right up the block from your home or you do not have to feel guilty that your husband or wife is training for a marathon. It is what it is!

Needless to say I've found a fitness plan that works just for me. I've found some supplements that work just for me. You will find a plan that will work just for you as well. This is what this book is about. Am I super thin, heck no! But I am getting fit. My blood pressure is great and so is my cholesterol. I have even dropped a few pounds. My doctor tells me to keep doing what I am doing and to tell you the truth that's all any of us can do.

CHAPTER TWO

MOTIVATION, COACHING, PHOOEY

I remembered when I received my Turbo Jam DVDs in the mail. I was so excited. I open the package and saw all the DVDs, the food guide and a jump start brochure. I read it from cover to cover and I put one of the DVDs in the DVD player. I went into the kitchen got me a slice of pepperoni pizza and my tall glass of ice cold Pepsi and proceeded to look at the DVD of the ladies and gentlemen doing their Turbo thing.

Don't get me wrong. I never plan on starting that day. I always start my fitness and diets routines on Monday (remember I told you this already) and I received my Turbo Jam on a Wednesday. But the entire time I was looking at the DVD I kept saying I can do that. It does not seem hard at all. When I tried the cardio DVD is was a killer workout. I truly enjoyed it. I continued to work out with the Turbo Jam crew for about 9 days. I bought Turbo Jam about 5 years ago and I still have 4 DVDs that I never saw. Wow!

My sister-in-law purchased the Yoga series for me for my birthday. I looked at the DVD like I normally do while having a snack and I did the one DVD exactly one time. I think it was called Windsor Pilates. I literally could not stretch my body to do any of the poses. I had that series for about seven years. Wow!

Oh, let us not forget the ball with that Gunnar guy and the lady that hosts Dancing with the Stars. I really enjoyed working out with this series. What's not to like? I am sitting down on a ball doing exercise. But then the fall lineup started and well everything changed after that. Goodbye, Brooke, goodbye ball, hello McDreamy! But I still have that ball in the guest room.

How many times have I seen Dr Phil, Oprah, Dr. Oz and magazines on the grocery line telling us about how this person lost a gazillion pounds? Here is how she/he did it and so can you! How many books do I have from Dr. Oz to Dr Atkins telling me to watch what I eat? Several and you know what, I still have the books and their methods did not make me lose the weight or want to get fit.

Do you remember going to a conference or seminar and you are gung-ho for the products and the people there were excited and got you all excited? You release your check book at the back of the room and bought their box of goodies because you are now equipped to do whatever they said you were suppose to do. But when you get home and you see all of the tapes, DVDs, pamphlets and flowcharts you start to feel blah about it. You no longer have that sitting on top of the world feeling like

> *Only you can motivate YOURSELF! Only you can decide to do whatever it is someone else is telling you to do.*

you had at the conference. You all know what I am talking about. Well, that is how I feel when I get anything coming in the mail about health and fitness. I am so pumped and excited looking at the commercial but when it is all said and done. I have just wasted my three easy payments of $29.99.

Only you can motivate YOURSELF! Only you can decide to do whatever it is someone else is telling you to do. Everything comes down to deciding to make a decision. If you are not ready believe you me you are not going to move.

The beauty of this book is simple. You will find your fitness and health program your way on your terms. It is okay to try something and then stop! You may have to talk to yourself. I do. For instance you can say I will do one sit-up at this time. If I do one today that is perfectly okay and I will celebrate doing that one. If you do not praise yourself for the one sit-up, you are going to have a hard time not only getting fit and healthy but in everyday decisions pertaining to your life. All we do is complain and murmur and murmur and complain and not grateful for the things we have already and for the things we can do at this very moment. If we left the murmuring and complaining out of our everyday conversation you will be amazed how our lives will turn around for the better.

The first time I did a superman (it looks so easy by the way) I think I did it for 3 seconds. Just try it. You lie on the floor, put both your hands out in front of you and lift your legs and arms out at the same time. Feel it baby. Wow! After doing the superman for 3 seconds I was so proud of myself. I probably can go a little longer now, but not by much. But the point is I did the superman for 3 seconds and I was proud. I did not say why I couldn't hold it longer, what is wrong with me or I am so out of shape. Do you when you are ready to do you!

I say forget about playing motivational tapes if you are just going to feel guilty because you have lost just 3 pounds but the person on the tape is telling you it should be 30 pounds. Who needs to feel bad like that? Then you wonder why you are not motivated anymore to continue. Stop! It is okay for someone to give encouraging words and thoughts. It is fine to have a coach for accountability and for guidance. But if you find yourself feeling more like a failure then a conqueror I say ditch the motivational tapes or the coach. Having a coach or listening to a tape should make you want to conquer whatever you need to conquer without making you feel like a failure. Never let another person make you feel like a failure! Remember there is absolutely nothing wrong with you. You just need to do things in a different way.

I do not listen to motivational tapes when it comes to fitness and health. I rather have a conversation with God. You can as well or not, it is simply up to you. I find that when I talk to Him I feel validated, wonderful and beautiful anyway. He does not create junk and we all are wonderfully and fearfully made. So with that mindset I do not need the tape. I strongly recommend having a conversation with God. He always listens and if you are quiet enough He will tell you that you are doing a terrific job and He is right there with you on the floor, couch, job or chair.

I say forget about playing motivational tapes if you are just going to feel guilty because you have lost just 3 pounds but the person on the tape is telling you it should be 30 pounds. Who needs to feel bad like that?

{CHAPTER THREE}
NOTHING NEW/ CHANGE OUR WAYS

If you think I am going to do the rundown of why we should all be fit and healthy, I am not. I am not going to discuss all of the diseases and ailments we are destined for if we do not get fit. I am not going to go over how obesity is a big problem in this country. We already know this. All we have to do is look in the mirror. All we have to do is listen to what the doctor said about our annual checkup. All we have to do is see how winded we are when we play with our children or grandchildren. All we have to do is see how tired we get when we are in the mall and can't visit all the stores because we are beat down. But I would like to discuss how we can change some of our ways.

Hear me out. I am not the authority on weight loss and fitness and Lord knows I do not pretend to be. One thing I know for sure I was thin and in pretty good shape playing handball and running around Manhattan from 34th street to the Village to find the perfect pair of shoes to being overweight and purchasing a blood pressure monitor machine. Believe me being fit is much better!

I wanted to write a little about my journey because you have the same journey when it comes to health and fitness. I did not tell you anything that I wouldn't tell my best friends Niecy and Tracy. Some of us are not the athletic type, or the healthiest, or have a career that we are constantly on the move. I wanted to address people like us for a change. The book is written in plain simple sentences and I am writing it as if I am talking to a person. If I didn't know something, I researched and found the answers. If I wanted to expound on something a little more I found the right person to help me. Sometimes you don't need to know it all but you should know how to find the person who does.

I know that most people gain weight and it is not until something happens that you realize that you have become over weight and unfit. Yes, you know you have gained weight but you do not realize you have become fat or almost unrecognizable. Let me explain. I did not gained 52 pounds all at once. It was an accumulation of living a sedentary life, contentment in my home and family and just being in a good place. Then one Thanksgiving weekend we all went to my uncle and aunt's house and we are having a good time and taking pictures and my little sister passed the camera over to me to look at the picture we just took less than 10 seconds ago and I literally did not know who that fat woman was, then it hit me, that was me!

We all have that moment. Now did I lose my mind and stop eating and ran for miles and all of this other stuff. No! I came to the conclusion that I am no longer thin, nor thick or even voluptuous. I am now fat! Now some people get a revelation and they begin a new fitness and health regime. I did that in my twenties. They are dedicated and they throw out everything in the kitchen and they tell everyone, hey, I am on a diet. Those types of people are what I call special.

Remember when I said we have to make a decision to decide to change something. Well let us revisit that statement. First of all you would not have purchase this book if you didn't want to try or do something else pertaining to your health and fitness.

So what if you are one of the hundreds of adults who suffer from chronic back pain. You may have gained weight simply because your mobility was limited. You probably were okay with that. Now you notice the weight gain is affecting your back even more and the doctor is concern this extra weight is having an adverse effect on healing. What are you going to change? What are you going to do?

You are an entrepreneur and have a home base business. You sit at your desk all day long. Is your office the dining room, right next to the kitchen? How convenient to run and get a snack quick fast. Is your office upstairs away from the kitchen but you tend to have the entire bag of chips or the entire bag of cookies upstairs so you do not have to keep going up and down the stairs? You have not taken a break from the computer screen in hours and you have been on the phone calling potential clients all day. You notice you have on sweat pants and they seem snug. Sweat pants, snug! What are you going to change? What are you going to do?

> *I could go on and on about how changes can be good. But notice all of these changes really do not apply to me or my life directly.*

You have worked all day long. Your boss got on your last nerve and your daughter still has not taken the clothes out of the dryer like you told her to do. You do not feel like cooking so you tell your son to order a pizza. You go to your bedroom thinking you are going to relax but all you do is stress about the things that have happened, the things that are happening and the things that will happened! Pizza's here. You have notice that you have not been cooking like you once did. It is so easy to tell the kids to get pizza or Chinese food. Your blood pressure is going up. Need to monitor that a little more. You eat your pizza and then you look at one of the housewives from somewhere on TV. You realize you do not feel so good. Heartburn, again? What is going

But when I make a change such as learn a new skill, learn how to plant a garden or how to conserve energy, what happens?

on? What are you going to change? What are you going to do?

Change can be good. I like Wendy's new fries with the sea salt. I like Bank of America has an app that I can check my balance at a moment notice on my iPod. I like that some companies really care about sustainability. I could go on and on about how changes can be good. But notice all of these changes really do not apply to me or my life directly. So what Wendy has new fries or Bank of America has an app for my iPod these things can happen or not and I will not gain anything from them. But when I make a change such as learn a new skill, learn how to plant a garden or how to conserve energy, what happens? I have educated myself in learning something new that can potentially increase my monetary value for my family or plant a garden to feed my family for months on end and save myself hundreds of dollars when I learn how to conserve energy. These changes produce positive results in my life. What do you think is going to happen when we sit at our desks, chairs or couches and do legs lifts or flex our arms or drink an ice cold seltzer water with 100% sugar free grapefruit juice? Yum! You will begin to see the stomach shrink; you will see the arms tightening and the legs becoming stronger. It does not have to happen in a month or even two but as long as something positive is happening.

One of the things this book can offer you is what to do while you are occupied doing something you enjoy. People like us need something different because if not we are quick to make an excuse. We are too quick to say my back is paining me so I better sit down until the pain subsides. I have a deadline, I need to stay at this desk and not move! What would people in the office say if they saw me doing a lunge at my desk? We have to stop and decide to make the decision that change is good and we do not have to be afraid.

One of the things this book can offer you is what to do while you are occupied doing something you enjoy. People like us need something different because if not we are quick to make an excuse.

Chapter Four

Food

My favorite food is Italian. I would love to go to Italy right now but I do not want to worry about how much I am eating, or what has this in it or that. I just want to eat and enjoy myself. I want to eat all the different pastas along with the many sauces. As I am writing this my mouth is watering for a piece of crusty bread dip in extra virgin olive oil along with some herbs. Ummm!

What can I tell you about food? We need it to live. We all have our favorite meals. But what makes us so crazy for food that we can become addicted to it or repulse by it? How can food have that type of power over us? I often wonder about that myself but I do know that food is doing a job on our children as well as adults. Obesity must be a big deal when the First Lady is asking Beyonce to do a video so the children can move.

I will admit we can make better choices and we will, when we decide to make the decision to change our eating habits. I will admit I am a carbohydrate, sugar/sweet/bread loving type of gal. But my eating habits were a bit much. Pepsi is my drink of choice. Ask all of my co-workers from the Wall Street days what I ate and drank for breakfast, a bialy (similar to a bagel but flatter and better) with bacon and eggs and a Pepsi. Maybe on a Friday I would add some home fries. Eating like this and going out every Thursday for drinks, wings and things began to change my body. The weight came on. You all know what I did. But of course I was really young and shallow and I just refuse to let my weight continue to escalate.

I still like these things but I just do not indulge all the time. I am going to let you in on some secrets of what I do which helps a lot. Now, before I go any further I am not telling you what brand of food you should be eating. I am not endorsing any type of food. I am just mentioning what I use and you can use that particular brand or you can use something similar. Pepsi or any other product is not giving me one red cent to mention them, but how are you going to know the changes I have made if I do not mention some of the products? Make sense, right?

Drinks

If you are a soda drinker and you have over 10 pounds to lose you have to ditch it. I know it hurts because Chinese food tastes so much better with Pepsi. Do not buy sugar free colas because they just make you mad because you really want the real deal and why have chemicals going into your body unnecessarily. But if you have to have a cola or Mountain Dew, Crush or anything bubbly, here is something you can do. Buy some seltzer water and add grapefruit juice or orange juice or any other type of juice as long as it is 100% sugar free. We all know that the juices are loaded with sugar and if I have to drink a juice with 28 grams of sugar I rather drink a Pepsi. It tastes like the Izze products. They are delicious but they can be pricey for a 4 pack.

Now if it is at all possible try to buy smaller seltzer waters because they do tend to go flat and what is the purpose of drinking them if we do not see the bubbles and hear the fizz. If you can find other drinking substitutions without chemicals and sugar you can drink that as well. But leave the soda alone.

If you like sweet tea or ice tea, add honey, a little lemon juice and nothing else. I can drink ice tea without sugar now and the flavor does not bother me as long as it is cold. You will be amaze of what your body will thank you for. I do not particularly like hot tea without sugar but I will drink it.

I also like drinking juices that are 100% sugar free. They have cherry, pomegranate and all sorts of other juices. You do not have to drink water at every meal although drinking water is cool.

For those of you who like coffee for breakfast you need to ditch the sugar and learn to drink it without. I cannot speak on Truvia or Stevia but maybe you could use them. If you notice any side effects immediately stop using them.

Milk is one of my favorite drinks as well. I drink the 1% or skim. But to tell you the truth my mother bought the 1% or 2% milk when we were kids and we were never wiser. If you do not have anything to drink in the house but you need something outside of water, milk is your choice.

Water is something we need or we die. Our body is practically all water. I like it but I am not in love with it. I am not convinced the flavor water or enhance water makes drinking water more pleasurable but whatever can get you drinking it, I guess is okay by me. I put lemons or lemon juice, water and ice into my personal blender and make a slushy. It can be sour but you can always add some type of fruit to it. It is so refreshing. You are drinking water and you are getting the added bonus of citrus which aids in blocking fat. So bring on the slushy. By the way you can get a personal blender for less than twenty dollars. A very handy appliance when you need to fix something up as soon as possible. When things are not easily accessible to some of us, we tend to do what? We order something we do not have any business ordering or we go into the freezer and get some processed food and put it in the microwave and call it a night. I know, I have the tee shirt, the hat, and the box to put it in. Having certain staples prepared saves a lot of headaches and pounds.

Fruits

What's not to like about fruit? It is sweet and taste good and refreshing. So why in the world we don't eat enough of it? I am guilty of having fruit go bad on me on several occasions. Can you believe that? How in the world can you let fruit go bad? Easy! You are eating what you really want to eat like the cookies, cakes and candy. Before you realize it the grapes look funny and the apples look bruise and scary.

One thing I recommend is when you purchase your fruit and bring them home, cut up the fruit. I hope you have plastic containers because they are going to be your best friend. Cut up your watermelon and cantaloupes in squares. If you have a nice decorative bowl, place apples, pears, bananas in the bowl on the kitchen table so you and everyone in the family can see it. It is real easy to grab an apple when you are going to sit down and do a little bit of reading. Sometimes you can put fruit into the crisper or the back of the refrigerator and forget you have them.

Now when you know you are craving something sweet and it is usually after dinner, don't look into the cabinet for some cookies or a Twinkie. Grab some of your fruit and put it in a bowl as if you were putting ice cream in the bowl. Leave the kitchen. It is imperative that you have cut up fruit in your refrigerator at all times. You make sure you have grapes (a variety), berries if in season, all the melons chopped. If you take them out of the grocery bag cut them up immediately. This method has save me many times. Believe me it hurts when you are losing weight and you do some dumb move and then get back on the scale and you see you have gained three pounds just that quick just because you had to eat 6 chocolate chips cookies or a candy bar or eat some potatoes chips, all because you didn't have anything cut up and prepared.

But it is okay. Sometimes we all want something chocolaty or sweet. You can eat a ton of fruit and that feeling just does not go away. Now, when that craving hits here is what I do. I am not telling you to do this because unfortunately not everyone has will power, but if you want to, buy some dark chocolate. No, they are not my favorite. I like milk chocolate but if I didn't like them so much I wouldn't be writing this book now, would I? You can eat two pieces which is enough to take away the craving and will not sabotage your diet if you do not go overboard.

Vegetables

I love most vegetables but the vegetables I don't particular care for, everyone seems to love. I can't stand string beans, carrots and cauliflower. I have tried to eat string beans every which way but I just do not like the flavor. Is it me or does carrots seem to be in every soup or frozen food entrée imaginable? Cauliflower is tasteless to me. You could put a pound of crispy bacon on it and it still wouldn't have any taste. Just my opinion people. You may love these vegetables or not but the point is we should be eating more of them.

The trick is when you buy your vegetables try to buy them frozen or fresh. The can stuff is okay but frozen and fresh seems to be tastier. Now if you are a snacker, a person who likes to nibble throughout the day then vegetables are your greatest bet for snacking. You see in a lot of diet books, it seems like vegetables are a get free card. You can eat a ton of it and it will not affect your diet. It is good for you and there is no limit. This information is according to some of the diet books I have accumulated throughout the years.

So when you come home with your peppers, carrots, celery, cherry tomatoes, etc, cut them up immediately and put them in a plastic bag or plastic container. If you want to snack on something the veggies are already cut up. If you are coming home and have to cook, if the vegetables are already cut up you can make a quick stir fry, quick stew, soup or side dish. It is all about having things done in advance so when you are lazy, in pain, aggravated, or running late, cooking dinner should not be a production. If you eat what you are supposed to eat you won't have to feel guilty again because you ordered the pizza or Chinese takeout.

Now if you look at the frozen section you see there are a ton of frozen meals vegetables such as corn, sweet peas, spinach, broccoli, etc. I usually save those for days I do not have any cut up vegetables. You just put them in the microwave add your sea salt or whatever seasoning you like along with your meat and you are good to go.

Now don't get sucked into buying those frozen dinners. You know the ones with chicken or beef with pasta and vegetables. They look so good on the package but when you take it home they don't taste all that good and they are loaded with salt. If we just cut back on salty foods we could weight ourselves and see a weight loss difference of 5 to 7 pounds. Don't even put it in the shopping cart.

Sometimes vegetables can be daunting because we are so set on eating the basic. I have learned to eat and love Bok Choy, squash and zucchini. Asparagus is my favorite vegetable. I have it at least three times a week. Yes, it is expensive but it is so good. I tried growing it but to no avail. I do not make any special sauce but I use sea salt, garlic and cracked black pepper with just a little extra virgin olive oil. I can't tell you how many people have tried my asparagus and they tell me they had no idea it tasted that good.

The key to eating different vegetables is simple. You have to know how to season them. You should have cracked black pepper, sea salt, olive oil, garlic, red pepper flakes, chicken stock and garlic powder. Play around with seasoning and you will notice that you will fall in love with most vegetables. Now I will understand if you don't fall in love with carrots, green beans or cauliflower. In my opinion no amount of seasoning can make these vegetables pop.

Beans and Legumes

If you are press for time beans bought in the can are fine. If they seem too salty just rinse them. You can do a lot with beans. I just go on the Internet and look for an exciting recipe for navy beans or pinto beans or whatever type of beans I have on hand. If you eat enough of beans you can even skip eating meat. I try to skip at least two days out of the week from eating meat. You have to do a little bit at a time. I notice when I try to implement all these dietary changes in one setting I failed horribly.

Some beans taste good in salads. They give that texture that helps especially when you are not trying to add bread crumbs to your salad. See some of us, not all don't have a problem eating a salad but we want to add so many unnecessary things on it that the calories add up tremendously. Please, if I am going to blow those types of calories it surely will not be with a darn salad!

Carbohydrates

Well what can I say about carbohydrates. To tell you the truth I notice when I cut down on them my stomach becomes flatter. I still like my pancakes and pasta. Now when I eat my pasta I just buy whole grain. It still tastes good to me.

I am a bread person but lately I have cut back on the everything bagel, biscuits and rolls. But I do allow myself one slice of honey wheat bread. Everyone in the family seems to like that bread the best as oppose to the 100% whole wheat bread.

Now as far as the starchy vegetables like corn, sweet peas, potatoes or sweet potatoes I still eat them but if I want French fries I bake them. I would suggest not having any frying oil in the house so you won't get tempted to fry anything.

Now, have I stopped eating fried foods? No, but I just don't fry it in my house. If I have a craving for fried chicken or fried fish I will purchase it outside my home. Maybe once a week or every 10 days or so I will have something fried and you know what I am okay with that. You will be surprise what you can do and what you can eliminate for a few days or even forever and be content with the decision. You may choose not to eat fried foods anymore and that is great. I am just not there yet.

Fats

I love having nuts and seeds around. I know you have to be careful of how much you're eating when it comes to nuts. But when I feel like something crunchy like chips or cookies I notice if I eat a few walnuts or pecans it really satisfies me. So when you feel like eating things that can jeopardize your weight loss efforts find some nuts and seeds such as pecan, walnuts, cashew, almonds, pumpkin seed, sunflower and of course peanuts. You may not like all of these so go to your favorite health food store and measure just a little bit of each for the ones you are not sure of. The reason for this is nuts can be pricey and the nuts and seeds at the health store are raw, without salt and seasoning. But they will take the edge off when you want to snack.

As far as oils I only use canola when it is in the house and Extra Virgin Olive Oil which I keep in my house. I sauté my vegetables with garlic and olive oil. It has a good flavor and I like how it makes the vegetables look silky and delectable. I am not the expert on which is the best oil to use but after looking at a ton of shows on cooking, reading books, magazines articles on healthy eating you really can't go wrong with olive oil.

{Chapter Five}

When TV Comes Before Exercising

Why do some of us hate the thought of exercising? Why do we make up any excuse not to do them? I truly do not know the answer to that question but here's a lists of excuses I have used and I have heard from others!

- *I don't want to mess my hair up.*

- *I am too tired to think about exercising.*

- *I don't like them because they are boring.*

- *I need the right clothes to exercise. As soon as I get some money I am going to buy the right outfit to exercise.*

- *I don't have time. I am way too busy.*

- *With my job, kids, spouse that is enough exercise for me.*

- *These exercises are way too hard for me.*

- *My game or my TV show is coming on.*

- *It is too late when I get home. I can't get up any earlier.*

- *Can't afford the gym.*

- *This neighborhood is too dangerous to walk around.*

- *I don't have the space in my apt or house.*

- *I have health problems.*

- *I might hurt myself.*

These are some of the most common excuses but I am quite sure there are many others.

I will be using the word "TV" as an example for anything in our lives that prevent us from exercising or moving.

Our TV could be our computer. We want to check out the latest on YouTube, do some online shopping, and catch up on homework or office work.

Our TV could be our friends. We hang out at the bar, check out the newest Denzel movie or just hang out at each other homes.

Our TV could be anything that distracts us from taking care of ourselves. I use to think why we just can't eat whatever we want and exercise when we feel like it and remain the same weight and still be fit and healthy as long as we are not over doing it. But folks it just does not work like that. Eating certain foods really do make us feel bad and sluggish. So if we are feeling sluggish what is really going on in the inside of our bodies? If we already have health challenges shouldn't we owe it to ourselves to put better things in our body?

Why not incorporate movement when we are dead set on our "TV" moments. For instance when you are actually looking at a show, do some type of exercise during the commercials.

When you are sitting at your computer, tell yourself that you will work for 15 minutes and then stop and *stop* and do some type of movement.

When you are hanging out with your friends tell them you need to do some type of movement. If they want to participate that is great, you never know how you may jumpstart something.

Believe it or not your friends know you are out of shape or not the healthiest person on the planet. Remember this is not news to anyone. Most of us just will not say anything unless it is totally out of control. So believe me they may be thrill that you are taking charge of your life.

When your TV is your family and you do everything for them and nothing for yourself you are heading for trouble. Get your entire family out for at least 15 minutes for some type of movement. I do not care where you live just move according to what you are capable of doing. You are with your family and they know. Your family knows before anyone else what you are going through. But when you put matters in your own hands and the family sees this they become excited as well. I am writing this stuff and in some weird way I am sounding just like the writers from the fitness books I have in my home. I hate it, but most of the things they are saying are dead on.

> *When your TV is your family and you do everything for them and nothing for yourself you are heading for trouble.*

Your job is your TV and you really have to draw the line somewhere. In between checking emails and making cold calls or whatever it is that you do make the time to do some type of movement.

Any type of movement is better than none. Doing something every day will help the body in more ways than one. I know it is hard but you can do something for your body even if you want to still do the "TV" thing first.

CHAPTER SIX

JUST FOR US

Do you know how you go to a salad bar and there are so many foods to choose from to make your salad just how you like it?

What about the all you can eat places? Even when you go on a cruise you have choices of what activities you can participate in. I like the idea of custom living. You may not want the same things I want, or do the same things that I want to do but that is okay because we can custom design our lives to fit us.

Why not a health and wellness plan? Each and every one of us has something going on in our lives that may make the same health and wellness program viable for others and not so for some. Wouldn't you want a program specifically for you to follow? Wouldn't you want a fitness expert to plan an exercise program for you with your back problems, arthritis pain or your sedentary life style? I would think so.

Why are these programs not readily available? Do the health and wellness industry feel this may not be a viable market? Do they not feel senior citizens want to be healthy and strong? How about the person who had surgery for cancer? Wouldn't they like to know about natural supplements and foods they could take to build their bodies up? What about the person who has always tried to be fit and now is newly diagnose with fibromyalgia or a condition that may change his/her mobility? Shouldn't there be a program for them as well?

All about Me Fitness is just a start. It will start out as a dialogue and hopefully begin to take shape and root. As more people with health problems, chronic pain, morbidly obese, sedentary life styles, and senior citizens begin to voice that they no longer want cookie cutter plans and they now want plans just for them, we will see doctors, physical therapist, wellness companies, fitness experts, trainers looking at the fitness market in an entirely new way.

All it takes is one person to address an issue. All it takes is one rally, one remark, one book, one radio station, one petition, one tweet, one person to say we need a change! How many people you know did not take care of themselves because they felt they had no choices? Now you do.

All about Me Fitness will start the dialogue. You will never be alone again in looking for something just for you. Yes, we have different programs and items showcase in this book but there are others out there.

We showcase a company that has oxygen on the go for when you need mental clarity or the strength to do something. How about when you are at your desk listening to a teleseminar or webinar, do you know you can juggle your way into fitness? What about simple techniques of breathing to lose weight? Hypnosis, anyone? We are talking about some innovative ways to get fit and healthy. Everyone loves chocolate, how about chocolate that helps you lose weight and gives you a jolt of energy.

I personally do not endorse any products, services, tools or exercise programs. You will have to do your due diligence. Ask the questions, tell them what you need, what you have, what you are willing to do or not. Make it personal because this is just for you. Ask, no demand exercises that are geared just for you. Ask the expert what you can do if you have other health conditions or you are a home base entrepreneur who sits all day. What about the morbidly obese, do you think they all want to have surgery? We need to know that we could be just as fit as the person who trains for the marathon or the person who can do P90X. We want the industry to take another look at us. We want to be taken serious. We want to see programs advertise on TV for us as well. We want good natural substances and a good solid exercise program as well.

As the author of this book I can honestly tell you I am thrill that we will see changes in the health and wellness world. But only if people like you begin to say

All it takes is one rally, one remark, one book, one radio station, one petition, one tweet, one person to say we need a change!

something. At your next wellness checkup ask your doctor if he/she knows of trainer who can help you with some moves since you have (fill in the blank). I know we all are living longer but we want to live happier lives. Yes, we may have obstacles and issues but we can live productive lives with what we have and what we are capable of doing right at the moment. Remember, murmuring and complaining never helped anyone.

All about Me Fitness will answers some questions that you never even ask before. I hope you begin a dialogue with some of the people who are anxiously waiting to answer any questions and concerns you may have. If you feel you need more, stay in touch. I will not rest until we have quality programs for all of us!

CHAPTER SEVEN

VITAMINS, TOOLS AND SUPPLEMENTS

This section contains different businesses that offer vitamins and supplements that will aid in the war on weight and having a healthier lifestyle. You know your body better than anyone else. Look at what they have to say about their product. If you feel it can aid you in getting fit by all means get in contact with them. Each and every representative list their name, email and web address so you can get in touch with them and ask for further information. Each section will go in details of exactly what the product will entail. My only criteria were the products had to be natural. Before taking any supplements ask your doctor first.

{ *You know your body better than anyone else. Look at what they have to say about their product.* }

{COCOA 101}

http://www.cocoa101.com

Diana McCalla

(949) 584-1630

www.cocoa101.com

Email: Diana@cocoa101.com

Chocolate, Free Radicals and Weight Control
{BY DIANA MCCALLA}

Behind the Science

It's no secret that obesity and unwanted weight gain is one of today's biggest health problems. A big component of the obesity problem is the free radical problem. Free radicals are "rogue" molecules that rob electrons from other molecules, which in turn become free radicals and "pinball" around the body, creating a continuous cycle of damage and destruction to our bodies' cells, tissue and organs.

Numerous studies demonstrate that free radicals lead to

unwanted weight gain. For instance, researchers from the Linus Pauling Institute at Oregon State University found a direct correlation between oxidative stress (free radical damage) and increased obesity. Another study from the University of Florida found that eating plants high in phytochemicals (and antioxidants) is effective at reducing the amount of oxidative stress in the body, and therefore able to lower the risk of gaining unwanted fat.

Other research suggests that chocolate also helps encourage weight loss in others ways. These include appetite suppression, healthy blood sugar maintenance, free radical control/antioxidant support, mood and craving control, boosts metabolism, relieves inflammation, increases energy and gene modulation.

Free Radicals Lead to Weight Gain

Researchers from the Linus Pauling Institute recently stated, "Obesity, as measured by body mass index (BMI), is independently associated with oxidative stress and confirms recent data." (Arteriosclerosis, Thrombosis, and Vascular Biology. 2003;23:365.)

The Antioxidant Solution to Weight Loss

As mentioned, free radicals are a major source of illness, aging and increasing health problems, including obesity. The good news is that eating a diet rich in antioxidants can be one of the best ways you can lose those unwanted pounds and improve overall wellness. Want to drop a few pant sizes? Want to lose inches off your waist, thighs and arms? Want to feel that surge of youthful energy? Want to have glowing skin? What about sharper mental focus, or improved sexual health? You can! And it's with a high-antioxidant or high-ORAC diet.

Finally, scientists and dietitians are talking about it, the mainstream media is reporting it and authors are writing books about it. There is a company that has harnessed the power of chocolate, and that is Xocai. Xoçai has understood the importance of antioxidants for a long time. All Xoçai products are tested for their ORAC score and certified by Brunswick Labs, an independent laboratory that certifies the ORAC content of foods and products for consumer education.

The good news is that Xoçai's healthy chocolate products are some of the highest ORAC products available today. And now, with the X-Protein Meal Replacement Shake—which boasts an amazing 50,000 ORAC score per serving—you can significantly boost your antioxidant intake and ORAC consumption and lose weight at the same time!

The High Antioxidant Wellness System

If you've searched for the answer to your weight loss woes, search no more. Xoçai's 30-day High-Antioxidant Wellness System is unlike any other system, helping you to lose weight, boost energy, feel great and improve overall wellness. Undoubtedly you've tried numerous programs or products before that yielded either unsatisfactory or temporary results. But this one won't, because researchers find that consuming 50,000 ORAC every day tends to produce the results you're looking for.

Based around the antioxidant-rich goodness of Xoçai healthy

chocolate, the X-Protein Meal Replacement shake delivers all the taste, nutrients and antioxidant firepower you'd expect from Xoçai—with only 190 calories and 50,000 ORAC per serving! And Xoçai offers other ORAC-rich healthy chocolate products as part of the system for added benefits.

With the Xoçai High-Antioxidant Wellness System, you will be eating at least 50,000 ORAC every day for the next 30 days (and we guarantee longer). Remember, the ORAC measures how well components of the food mop up the free radicals in the bloodstream. Eating 50,000 will boost the antioxidant potency of your blood at least 25% and provide additional weight loss firepower as well. This is one of those rare areas of nutrition where more truly is better.

What's In the Xoçai X Protein Meal Replacement Shake?

Below are just a few of the premium-grade ingredients in the X Protein Shake:

Cacao

- Is real, true cacao-based product – not simply "chocolate flavored"

- One of nature's top antioxidant super foods

- Proven to promote weight loss

- Protects heart, brain, GI tract, and other body systems

Whey Protein Isolate

- Can help promote healthy blood sugar levels

- Stimulates production of two appetite suppressing hormones

- Contains leucine, which promotes fat loss

Cocoa Fiber

- Promotes healthy digestion and elimination

- Is only product with cocoa fiber as primary fiber source

- Promotes satisfaction, suppresses appetite

Apple Fiber

- Helps promote feeling of satiety

- Supports healthy blood sugar/insulin levels

19 Amino Acids

- Are the building blocks of protein

- Assist in energy metabolism

- Enable vitamins, minerals, antioxidants and other nutrients to perform their duties

Acai Berry

- Boasts extremely high ORAC score

- Contains amino acids, essential fats and other healthful nutrients

Chia Seed Oil

- Is rich in omega-3 fats

- Helps promote cleansing

Xylitol

- Is an effective sweetener to standard sugars

Vitamins and Minerals

- 12 vitamins, including B vitamins for brain and appetite control

- 13 minerals, including chromium, manganese and zinc for weight control

Why Chocolate?

As the only cacao-based, high-antioxidant wellness product, the Xoçai X-Protein Meal replacement shake is in a class of its own. Numerous studies show cacao and healthy chocolate can help boost weight loss and increase overall wellness for various reasons:

- Is one of nature's top antioxidant foods

- Optimizes production of brain chemicals such as serotonin

- Decreases appetite

- Stabilizes blood sugar levels

- Improves mood

- Decreases inflammation

- Protects against stress and anxiety

10 Reasons to Use the Xoçai High Antioxidant Wellness System

The First and Only High-Antioxidant Product- Is the cornerstone of the High-Antioxidant Weight Loss system, which is the only cacao-based high-antioxidant product available, and is proven to promote weight loss.

The Original Healthy Chocolate- Contains the same revolutionary ingredients and nutrients that comprise Xoçai's healthy chocolate.

Unmatched Formulation- Contains the finest-source, whey protein isolate (20 g; 90% protein; quick cold water dispersion; highly digestible; low-glycemic; low-lactose, excellent amino profile), high-fiber blend of cocoa fiber and apple fiber, acai berries, blueberries, chia seed (an amazing nutrient-rich, omega-3 source), a blend of low-glycemic, low-sugar sweeteners¬—fruit sweet, xylitol, and sucralose (as a flavor enhancer), and fortified with vitamins and minerals, probiotics and 19 amino acids for not only enhanced weight control, but also a wide array of health benefits

ORAC Superstar- Delivers a mind-boggling 25,000 ORAC in every serving No Health Limitations. Is lactose-free and gluten-free

Perfect Balance- Contains 20 g protein, 3 g fats, 10 carbs, 2 g sugars, 8 g fiber, 19 amino acids and 0 g cholesterol.

Low-Calorie Superstar- Contains only 130 calories per shake!

It's Delicious. Delivers the same superior flavor of other Xoçai healthy chocolate products and provides a rich decadent chocolate taste of true cacao. Also enhances the rich cocoa flavor with acai, blueberries and other natural sweeteners.

It's Economical. Allows you to simply replace the $5 fast-food, super-sized meals that got you fat in the first place. By using this system, you will help eliminate the cost of hundreds of dollars worth of other unhealthy, high-calorie, empty-nutrition junk foods you normally purchase.

It's Convenient. Making the X-Protein Meal replacement shake is simple, fast and easy. Can be taken and made just about anywhere.

Is a Nutrient Powerhouse- Getting the 25000 ORAC score is easy and convenient with the X-ProMeal shake. You can get the full health benefits of multiple high-ORAC fruits, vegetables (example: 1 shake has the ORAC equivalent of 3 artichokes, 8 oranges and 50 cups of spinach) and other whole foods in just one X-Protein Meal shake, all without the additional carbs and sugars.

{SLIM & SASSY}

http://www.OilEssentials.org

Joni Lang

(480) 209-9639

www.OilEssentials.org

Email: jtlang1029@yahoo.com

Slim & Sassy Metabolic Blend

dōTERRA's Slim & Sassy Metabolic Blend is a proprietary formula of 100% pure CPTG Certified Pure Therapeutic Grade® essential oils designed to help manage appetite between meals. Slim & Sassy includes a blend of grapefruit, lemon, peppermint, ginger, and cinnamon essential oils. Just add 8 drops to 16 oz. of water (regular size bottle of water) and drink between your healthy meals throughout the day to help manage hunger calm your stomach, and lift your mood. The Slim & Sassy blend also makes delicious and healthy flavored water for proper hydration during exercise and other activity. It has zero calories and is an excellent replacement for high-calorie beverages or for drinks that contain artificial sweeteners and colors.

Primary Benefits

Supports your efforts to eat less and exercise more for permanent, healthy weight loss by helping your body adjust to reduced caloric intake during dieting.

Helps manage appetite and hunger pangs between meals*

Helps calm stomach and gastrointestinal distress sometimes associated with dieting*

Lifts and elevates mood which has been associated with successful weight-loss efforts

Encourages healthy hydration during dieting, exercise, and throughout the day*

What Makes This Product Unique?

Proprietary blend of 100% CPTG Certified Pure Therapeutic Blend® essential oils

No caffeine or other stimulants

No sugars, zero calories

No artificial colors, flavors, or ingredients

Easy and safe to use with no harmful side effects

Directions for Use

Add 8 drops of Slim & Sassy Metabolic Blend to 16 oz. of water. Sip your flavored water before, between, and after each of your healthy meals throughout the day. Slim & Sassy also makes an excellent addition to water bottles or hydration packs during exercise and outdoor activity. Slim & Sassy can be used aromatically by diffusing in your home or personal office space or by simply applying a few drops to the palms, then cupping your hands and breathing deeply for a moment of calm and meditation as you reprogram your body to your new healthy lifestyle.

Caution

Slim & Sassy is safe to use aromatically, topically or internally when used as directed. Because it contains citrus essential oils that may increase photosensitivity in the skin, it is recommended that you avoid sunlight or UV rays for up to 12 hours after topical application. Do not use directly in eyes, ears, or nose. Keep out of reach of children. If pregnant or under a doctor's care, consult your physician.

The Slim & Sassy blend also makes delicious and healthy flavored water for proper hydration during exercise and other activity. It has zero calories and is an excellent replacement for high-calorie beverages or for drinks that contain artificial sweeteners and colors.

SKINNY FIBER

Name: Sally Shields

Web address: www.sjcion.skinnyfiber.com

Phone number: (718) 543-5524

Email: blurbradio@gmail.com

Scientifically formulated with some of the world's healthiest ingredients, Skinny Fiber is WAY more than just another weight loss pill. Not only can Skinny Fiber help you feel full and eat less, but the Skinny proprietary blend when combined with healthy diet and exercise also help support weight management, metabolism, and a host of other benefits to your body.

Packed with our proprietary blend of ingredients, Skinny Fiber is not only designed to help support your weight loss goals, but also to support other healthy functions in your body. What if you could eliminate the #1 enemy of weight loss...overeating? With all natural dietary fiber Glucomannan, Skinny Fiber may be able to help. Glucomannan is a unique all natural soluble dietary fiber defined on Wikepedia as "a food additive used as an emulsifier and thickener."

Believed to expand in your stomach to make you feel full, Glucomannan may help suppress your appetite to overcome the #1 enemy to weight loss, overeating and cravings. In addition to the potential weight supporting benefits, in double blind clinical studies, Glucomannan has been shown to have other health benefits such as supporting healthy cholesterol levels and more. Glucomannan is a true wonder ingredient!

Carralluma, the Natural Appetite Suppressant! Caralluma is a plant, in the cactus family, that has been used as a natural appetite suppressant in India for centuries particularly in times of famine. "It is also used for its purported ability to suppress hunger and appetite and enhance stamina.

It is believed to have an effect on the appetite control centre of the brain." – Wikipedia Chá de Bugre - The Brazilian Secret Along the coast of Rio De Janeiro, Brazil, beauty is defined by how you look in a bikini. And one of the favorite ingredients used in beachfront restaurants and refreshment stands is Chá de Bugre...one of the key ingredients in Skinny Fiber.

In addition to being used as an appetite suppressant, Chá de Bugre may also support a healthy metabolism. In fact, it is brewed in large drums at times of festival in Brazil, so that people can drink it to sustain their energy. Another great benefit of this exciting ingredient!

 Much more than just another weight loss product, Skinny Fiber is formulated unlike ANY other product on the market. If you've tried other weight loss or diet programs, Skinny Fiber might be EXACTLY what you've been looking for! The perfect product for both men and women!

*Sally Shields is an award-winning pianist, composer, speaker, author and radio personality. Co-host of the exciting new BlogTalkRadio show, "Blurb!" Shields is a frequent contributor to various magazines, and has been featured in Star Magazine, Obvious, My Day, Girlfriendz, For the Bride and many others. Endorsed by Dr. Laura Schlessinger and Martha Stewart, she has appeared on Fox and Friends, and is a repeat guest on the nationally syndicated The Daily Buzzwith her Wedding Showers #1 Amazon.com bestseller, **THE DAUGHTER-IN-LAW RULES!** and her newest release on Blooming Twig Books, Is She Naturally Thin, or Disciplined? **INSIDER SECRETS of the SEXY and SLIM!***

What if you could eliminate the #1 enemy of weight loss...overeating?

TRIM ENERGY

www.togobrands.com

Company is To Go Brands – Product is Trim Energy™

www.togobrands.com

858-200-0678

inventivepr@att.net

All-natural Trim Energy™ is packed with healthy weight loss supporting nutrients to give you a Triple Action Edge to stick to your ALL-NATURAL weight loss plan! ***Action 1!*** Burn fat with the lean, green coffee bean! ***Action 2!*** Rev up metabolism with potent Green Tea! ***Action 3!*** Stress-less with the help of the Ashwagandha Herb!

Green Tea Energy Fusion is more than just tea. It is a fusion of healthy, all natural green teas and energizing herbs & extracts from around the globe. It is scientifically formulated to support the metabolism* and to give you the fuel you need to energize your body & refresh your senses. Organic Japanese Green Tea rich in EGCG 100 mg per serving has been added to this energizing formula to maximize metabolism support* and provide you with even more healthy EGCG antioxidants!

* L Theanine- A health optimizing amino acid that helps prevents the jitters.
* Organic Yerba Maté & Guaraná Seed Extract - Indigenous to South America, Yerba Mate has traditionally been used as a brewed drink for mental & physical fatigue. Guaraná has long been a popular ingredient in beverages in South America.
* Organic Aloe Vera- Called the Plant of Immortality by the ancient Egyptians; Aloe has been shown in some scientific studies to help the liver convert fats into energy.
* Siberian Ginseng- An adaptogen that can help increases the body's resistance to stress and support energy levels, Siberian Ginseng can also be helpful for reducing high blood sugar levels that often spike after meals.
*A combination of 90 mg of EGCG and 50 mg of Caffeine 3 times daily have shown metabolism boosting effects in clinical studies. A.G. Dulloo, American Journal of Clinical Nutrition, Dec. 1999

Green Tea Energy Fusion is more than just tea. It is a fusion of healthy, all natural green teas and energizing herbs & extracts from around the globe.

FRUIT ADVANTAGE

Traverse Bay Farms / Fruit Advantage

www.traversebayfarms.com

877-746-7477

Email: andy@traversebayfarms.com

The Triple Benefits of the Tart Cherry:
Help relief joint pain, help with gout and reduce belly fat.

The tart cherry offers a natural anti-inflammatory benefit not found in any other fruit. In fact, according to research from Michigan State University the Montmorency tart cherry offers 10 times the anti inflammatory benefits of OTC products including aspirin.

In addition, the tart cherry is a natural source for Cox-1 and Cox-2 inhibitors. This means the Montmorency tart cherry helps to block pains signals in the body. However, unlike prescription drugs it helps to protect the stomach from damage. Tart cherry concentrate is a highly concentrated way to get the natural pain fighting properties of the tart cherry juice.

It takes 60 -80 cherries to make just one ounce of the tart cherry juice concentrate. One reliable source for tart cherry juice concentrate is Traverse Bay Farms. http://www.traversebayfarms.com In addition to offering tart cherry juice concentrate, the company also offers tart cherry capsules, dried tart cherries and even organic tart cherries.

The tart cherry has also been shown to help lower uric acid in the body. The anthocyanins in this ruby red fruit are the compounds believed to help the body dissolve the painful crystals that form between the joints.

Finally, according to research from University of Michigan, a study of tart cherry powder fed to mice in the study had a positive effect on belly fat.

> *The tart cherry offers a natural anti-inflammatory benefit not found in any other fruit.*

FREEKAH

Barbara Incognito Fanelli

www.Freekehlicious.com

201-297-7957

Email: Freekehlicious@gmail.com

Freekeh (pronounced free-ka) is a new super food and ingredient. It is 'roasted green grains.' Freekeh is a process and not the name of a grain variety.

Freekeh is 100% natural! The grains are harvested while still soft, young and green, then parched, roasted and dried. The process captures and more importantly retains the grains at the state of peak taste and nutrition. Green grains are very different in properties to mature grains. The entire process is natural and only uses fire and air. No additives or preservatives are used. Freekeh is free from GMO.

Freekeh is considered to have low glycemic index with an excellent insulin response - good for preventing and managing diabetes. Freekeh is also high in "resistant starch."

Some studies indicate that resistant starch (which acts more like a fiber than a carbohydrate) may play a role in weight management - making it an excellent food for weight loss. And, because the grains are harvested while still young, freekeh retains more protein, fiber, vitamins, and minerals compared to traditionally processed wheat.

Health Benefits:

• Low carbohydrates, high in fiber (up to four times the fiber of brown rice). (CSIRO) Comparative Analysis between Freekeh, Rice and Pasta

• Acts as a prebiotic, fueling the growth of healthy bacteria in our digestive tract. (CSIRO)

• Low GI food with excellent insulin response. Good for preventing and managing diabetes. (CSIRO Report: Freekeh Composition and Glycemic Index Study.)

• Rich in lutein and zeaxathin — important phytonutrients for eye health and implicated in the prevention of age-related mascular degeneration. (University of Adelaide)

•Increases concentration and excretion of butyrate which is associated with diminishing the risk of developing colorectal cancer and diverticulitis (CSIRO Executive Summary: Effects of Freekeh on Biomarkers of Bowel Health and Cardiovascular Health.)

•Good for general bowel health. Beneficial for preventing constipation and managing Irritable Bowel Syndrome (CSIRO)

{ULTIMATE LIVING}

Ruthie Smith

www.ultimateliving.com

Email: ruthie@ultimateliving.com

(214) 252-2305 Direct Line

"Green Miracle" is a 100% natural live whole food. Three scoops provide you with 8,000 mg of pure nutrition, plus your daily requirement of fruits, veggies, and then some!

Green Miracle contains essential vitamins, minerals, amino acids, lignans, fiber, chlorophyll and enzymes. It assists in regulating your body's pH balance, helps to maintain proper glucose levels, stabilizes the metabolism, provides much needed energy and gives a powerful boost to your immune system. It contains over 80 different ingredients. It contains no added sugars and is safe for individuals taking glucose regulating prescriptions. After testing by the Diabetes Resource Center, Ultimate Living's Green Miracle was awarded the SEAL of APPROVAL as a beneficial food acceptable for diabetic consumption.

{CRAZY FOR NUTRITION}

Annemarie McDermott

www.crazyfornutrition.com

303.594.7466

Annemarie@crazyfornutrition.com

If you could change one thing about your diet, what would that be? Interested in shedding pounds, promoting anti-aging, boosting your immune system and preventing chronic disease such as cancer, diabetes and cardiovascular disease? Eating a diet rich in fruits, vegetables and grains is imperative to not only a healthy lifestyle but a balanced nutritious diet. It is recommended that we eat 9-13 servings (2011) of fresh fruits & vegetables EVERY DAY! Even with our best intentions, we lack the nutrients that our bodies so desperately need! Juice Plus+ is the *next best thing* to fruits & vegetables. With over 50,000 phytonutrients working synergistically together, your body is getting 17 different fruits, vegetables and grains DAILY at a fraction of the cost!

Juice Plus+ is NOT a supplement, it is whole food based nutrition made from fresh, high quality fruits & vegetables, carefully tested to ensure that no pesticides or other contaminants affect the natural purity of the product. It is kept at low temperatures to ensure all the nutritional value of the fruits & vegetables are not destroyed.

Juice Plus+ is backed by independent clinical research! With over 18 independent, third party, peer review published research conducted by many prestigious institutions throughout the world; it is one of the most thoroughly researched brand name nutritional products on the market today.

Children (ages 4-18 or in college) can receive their Juice Plus+ for FREE for up to 3 years when an adult is taking Juice Plus+. Through the CHILDREN'S HEALTH STUDY, we are seeing great improvements on family health!

I would love to see how Juice Plus+ can change your life as it has so many people around the world. Call for additional information or to get you started!

Juice Plus+ is the next best thing to fruits & vegetables. With over 50,000 phytonutrients working synergistically together, your body is getting 17 different fruits, vegetables and grains DAILY at a fraction of the cost!

www.mirafit.com

Name: Dr. Joseph Artiss and Dr. Catherine Jen

(248) 366-0388

Email: info@mirafit.com

What is Mirafit fbcx?

Mirafit fbcx is a soluble fiber derived from corn that reduces the absorption of dietary fat. One gram (one tablet) of Mirafit binds nine grams or 81 calories of fat. Six tablets per day prevent the absorption of a significant portion of the fat in a typical daily diet. In combination with a healthy diet and exercise program, use of this naturally occurring food supplement has been shown in clinical studies to support weight loss and to maintain healthy blood cholesterol levels. Mirafit is heart-friendly because it is stimulant- free.

The All- Natural Weight Loss Supplement, Mirafit fbcx, was developed by Wayne State University Professors Dr. Catherine Jen and Dr. Joseph Artiss. When taken as directed (2 pills with every meal), Mirafit can safely bind and remove 9 grams of dietary fat or 81 fat calories, which could add up to the loss of one to one and a half pounds every week. The supplement is derived from non allergenic corn fiber and has been granted a GRAS (Generally Regarded As Safe) Rating from the FDA.

OXYGEN ENRICHED AIR

Barbara Turner

www.EnergyNaturalway.com

202-436-5031

Email: oxygenlife4u@gmail.com

Previously only available to Elite Pro Athletes or by Prescription or to the super wealthy, the inventor of the Paintball craze brings the world the First Personal, Portable Oxygen in a Can! Safe for Students to Seniors...

Oxygen is the most important nutrient to the cells in your body. You can live without foods for weeks, without water for days and a few minutes without oxygen.

95% Oxygen Enriched Air is one of the fastest, most effective ways to flood your body with valuable oxygen!

- Non Prescription

- Convenient and Easy to Use

- Enters bloodstream in Seconds

- No Harmful Side Effects

- No Sugars, No Calories

- No Stimulants, No Crashing

Great for:

- Hangovers

- Seniors

- Altitude Sickness

- Stress

- Mental Clarity and Focus

- General Vitality

- Power and Endurance

- Speed and Quickness

- Training Intensity

- Recovery

Waiver: True Oxygen Enriched Air is NOT FOR MEDICAL USE and it is not intended to treat, cure or prevent diseases.

CHAPTER EIGHT

EXERCISES

We have fitness experts who have different methods of getting you in shape according to what you are capable of doing. Some are a little different than what you may be accustomed to seeing or doing. You have choices. As more people ask their doctors or talk to more health and wellness representatives about exercise programs geared for them we will begin to see a trend for customize programs.

Exercise is movement. You may not be able to move your left arm like you once could but maybe you can move other parts of your body. You may be slow in moving your entire body but yet you can still move but in a different way. You may have to sit down but you can still move your upper body and even your legs while sitting down. The key is to move your body each and every day deliberately.

Once you find the exercise plan that works best for you please inform your doctor first before trying any new exercise routine. Hopefully you will see a plan for you and if not other programs may become available that will be a fit for you.

 The following fitness experts will briefly talk about how their program helps and give some exercises you can try. I strongly urge you to get in touch with them for further information and clarification. They may be able to custom fit a plan just for you!

WEIGHT LOSS MINDSET

www.TheWeightLossMindset.com

Dr. Randy Gilchrist

(916) 899-4990

Email: drgilchrist@theweightlossmindset.com

I (Dr. Randy Gilchrist) am a clinical psychologist and hypnosis for weight loss expert in private practice in Roseville, CA (www.dr-rg.com). I am also the creator of The Weight Loss Mindset audio hypnosis program (www.TheWeightLossMindset.com). I myself have lost and kept off 70 pounds through hypnosis. Even though weight loss is the main issue people come in to receive hypnosis for, they also come in for a number of other addiction or anxiety related issues. I've been helping people as a psychotherapist for nearly 15 years.

Regarding The Weight Loss Mindset, it includes 8 hypnosis sessions addressing all of the main areas people would like help with to lose weight, including sessions to promote eating less, eating better, exercising more, avoiding junk food, etc. The program is powerful, effective, convenient, all-natural. You just listen whenever you have the time to relax and focus, such as just before going to bed. Then with practice, notice your motivation, focus, and commitment increase to finally follow through with your weight loss plan. Get your mind in line to lose weight! Come check it out on my website: www.TheWeightLossMindset.com, which includes a 60-second video introduction.

What is hypnosis? What if I can't be hypnotized/what if hypnosis doesn't work for me?

The process of clinical hypnosis is as follows: a subject closes their eyes, relaxes, and gets into a focused mental state (known as a trance) through the suggestions of a hypnotherapist. Then, the subject is given a number of suggestions for positive change which become easier to accept (now that conscious resistance is lowered).

This hypnosis process works well for most people (assuming the hypnotherapist is properly trained and experienced). It's important to know that "being strong willed" doesn't make it harder to be hypnotized. Neither does having a certain personality or having most learning disorders. Modern clinical hypnosis (like with this program) simply requires being able to relax and focus on what is being said for a stretch of time. If you can do those two things, then you can be hypnotized and benefit from hypnosis. This skill of being able to relax and focus is natural and doable for most people, becoming easier and stronger with time and practice.

I don't really like to exercise. Can hypnosis help me exercise more?

Yes. In fact, I've also devoted 3 of the 8 hypnosis sessions to the theme of exercising more and leading a more physically active lifestyle. Listening to these 3 sessions in particular ("enjoying exercise", "living an active lifestyle", and "getting the perfect body") will help you desire and engage in more exercise, as well as live a more active lifestyle in general.

JUGGLE FIT

Heather Wolf

http://jugglefit.com

850-932-5570

Email address: info@jugglefit.com

JuggleFit LLC provides products and resources that help people fit exercise and healthy eating into their busy schedules. By providing portable, effective ways for working out the body and brain as well as tools to facilitate healthy and easy-to-prepare food choices, JuggleFit makes fitness simple and fun. Juggling is one of the few cardio exercises that can be done while sitting in a chair, which makes it perfect to do during TV commercials or when recovering from a lower body injury. JuggleFit's recently released office fitness accessory, Cardio in a Box, brings the workout straight to the desk, with simple and light cardio, resistance and stretch moves that can be done throughout the workday.

Juggling is a truly portable workout

The equipment required for juggling is minimal and portable. Juggling scarves or balls fit into your purse, briefcase, backpack or luggage. And you can juggle in large or small spaces. This makes it the perfect exercise for business travelers, or anyone who finds themselves on the road- touring musicians, athletes, adventurers, campers, etc. Juggling is aerobic exercise, as long as you remember to BREATHE while doing it! It may be one of the few (or only) aerobic exercises you can do in a tiny space. You don't even need floor space if you juggle over a bed or couch!

It makes you smarter

Yes, it's true - juggling has been proven to increase the amount of gray matter in the brain (Nature magazine, volume 427, Jan. 2004). Research also suggests it may prevent Alzheimer's disease. When you juggle, you're not only burning calories, toning your body and strengthening your core, you're exercising your mind as well. This is why there's no need to worry about how long it takes you to learn how to juggle - you're still burning calories and boosting your brainpower. In fact, the longer it takes you to learn, the more you are exercising your mind!

Juggling sharpens focus & concentration

Juggling engages your problem-solving skills. You can't just throw all the balls up in the air and hope everything comes together! This is why juggling is excellent for helping you master the art of concentration. The intense focus required for juggling can filter into other areas of your life that require the same type of close attention.

Juggling is the ultimate in stress relief

When you are learning to juggle, you are immediately absorbed in the activity. It's almost impossible to think of anything but the task at hand. This makes it a great way to escape any worries, stress, hardships, or anything that might be hanging over your head.

Say you are overwhelmed with so much at work that you can barely think straight. If you pick up the juggling balls or scarves for as little as 5 minutes and practice, you will clear your mind and be able to tackle your job with more clarity and focus.

This effect is truly amazing. JuggleFit classes open with some discussion on juggling. Usually we can tell that some of the students are still thinking about the traffic jam they encountered on the drive in, or the grocery list they must fill after the class. But the minute we hand out those juggling scarves and begin to teach, every student is fully absorbed in the moment. We ask them if they are able to think about anything else, and they laugh and say 'no way'!

Juggling truly is one of the quickest ways to take your mind off something, which makes it the perfect form stress relief.

It doesn't feel like exercise

Many people are surprised to find out that juggling is exercise, and that is burns 280 calories per hour, much like walking. This is probably because it is so very different from running on a treadmill, lifting weights, or doing crunches or pushups. Simply put, these exercises do not make you laugh, and they are not usually entertaining to watch, unless you are attending bodybuilding competitions or the like. But juggling definitely makes you laugh, and is entertaining for others to watch, even if you are just learning! What other exercise has that effect? At JuggleFit classes, we always look forward to that first wave of laughter when everyone first tries to juggle.

You can juggle where you are, no travel required!

Let's face it, sometimes hitting the gym or going for that long run seems like an impossible wall to climb. Our bodies need a break from exercise, this is normal. Have you ever driven to the gym, started to workout and then realized your body was not up to it? Juggling is especially great for those times you may not be feeling up to a workout. It requires no time investment - you don't have to spend money on gas to drive to the gym, or waste that 15 minutes getting to the running trail. You can just pick up the balls and start to juggle. If your body is truly not up for exercise, you can just stop and there you are. No wasted time or gas money!

Juggling maintains and increases range of motion in the arms and shoulders

Juggling utilizes body mechanics in which we normally do not engage. It's great to move the body in new ways to maintain range of motion. The expression 'use it or lose it' applies here. Juggling lubricates the joints in the arms and shoulders, and keeps them from getting creaky as we age! That also makes juggling a great form of senior fitness for the same reason.

Juggling is one of the best ways to improve coordination

Many people say they can't juggle because they are too uncoordinated. Nine times out of ten, the people that say that are the first ones in the class to be able to juggle, no joke!

Even if you are truly uncoordinated, that's even more reason to add juggling to your fitness routine. Better coordination will make your daily activities easier and help prevent trips and falls (especially important for senior fitness). No one is able to juggle out of the womb. It takes practice! Remember that the act of learning how to juggle still burns calories, tones your body and boosts your brainpower.

You don't often hear about coordination as an essential element of overall fitness, but it is. And this is very interesting - JuggleFit has taught many athletes how to juggle, and they usually learn very quickly. Many are juggling balls in under 5 minutes. This makes perfect sense. Someone that must connect a racquet to ball, catch or hit a speeding baseball, or shoot into a basket for a living has developed a high level of coordination. As a result, juggling comes easy. This is not to say that coordinated athletes cannot benefit from juggling - quite the contrary. By learning more challenging juggling patterns and moves, they can take their coordination to even higher levels. There is no ceiling with juggling - there will always be something even the best juggler in the world cannot do!

You don't often hear about coordination as an essential element of overall fitness, but it is.

FIT DECK

Phil Black

www.fitdeck.com

858-453-6644

Email address: phil@fitdeck.com

FitDeck creates custom Exercise Playing Cards that make exercise, nutrition, and training for sports more simple, convenient, and fun.

About FitDeck Exercise Playing Cards

Q: What is FitDeck?

A: FitDeck is a unique deck of exercise playing cards containing illustrations and instructions describing different exercises, stretches, and movements. Our current line of 37 different FitDeck titles range from FitDeck Pilates to FitDeck Navy SEAL.

Q: What's the best way to use FitDeck cards?

A: There are hundreds of ways to use FitDeck cards depending on your fitness level, motivation, and resources available to you. The most basic way is to warm up, shuffle the cards, select a card, perform the exercise, and repeat as desired.

Q: How many cards should I start out with?

A: It depends on a number of factors: ability, age, fitness level, etc. An average person may choose to start off with five cards and then assess how they feel the next day. To be safe, most people begin using FitDeck cards every other day in order to allow for recovery time in between workouts. More advanced users may choose to begin with 15 – 20 cards in their first workout.

Q: Where do I find out about new FitDeck games and workout ideas?

A: Visit the FitDeck Workouts section of this website, which categorizes games and routines according to personal profiles. You can also purchase the Games & Activities Booklet, which contains over 70 different games and activities to use with FitDeck. You will also find a sampling of games and workouts on the Information Cards included in your FitDeck. Sign up for our newsletter which provides the latest workout tips, favorite routines, and new titles.

Q: Who will benefit from FitDeck?

A: People from age 5 to 85 years old can benefit from performing basic FitDeck exercises as long as they are taking into account their own personal abilities and limitations. It is always advisable to speak with your healthcare provider before beginning any new exercise program. It is well known that regular bouts of basic exercises and stretching will greatly improve your overall fitness and health.

Q: What makes FitDeck special?

A: FitDeck is special because it is simple, convenient, and fun. There are hundreds of workout routines and programs out there. Unfortunately, not many of them take into consideration the challenges that most people face trying to fit exercise into their daily lives. FitDeck is special because it recognizes these obstacles and does its best to work through them with a simple and user-friendly product.

ISOBREATHING

Ellen Miller

www.isobreathing.com

972-672-5381

Email address Ellen@isobreathing.com

IsoBreathing is known as the "Kindergarten" of exercise. Everyone needs a starting place. If you can BREATHE and you can SIT IsoBreathing will get you FIT!

IsoBreathing® is a combination of isometrics and slow, rhythmic breathing.

An isometric is a muscle contraction in which the tension increases, but the muscle length remains the same. Energy is expanded and calories burned by maintaining the contraction.

The breathing portion of IsoBreathing® is a specialized breathing that delivers oxygen to every part of the body being exercised. The breathing is slow and rhythmic.

Unlike some programs, with IsoBreathing® there is absolutely NO breath holding. Holding one›s breath, especially while exercising, can lead to lightheadedness and loss of consciousness.

No funny faces, no snorts or grunts, no calorie counting or diets involved - just smarter, healthier choices and low key resistance training. This slow rhythmic breathing can be done in public!

IsoBreathing

What is Isobreathing® and who can benefit from the program?

Who is the program designed for?

• Those who want to lose weight and inches starting with your first week.

• Those who want to learn to work their muscles without becoming sore

• Those that have physical limitations

• Those that do not work out on a regular basis

• Those who have tried it all without success

• Senior Citizens

I designed this program with my clients in mind. 75% of my clients need to lose anywhere from 35 pounds on up. From that group, more than half need to lose more than 100 pounds. You need to start somewhere and when you are morbidly obese you do have physical limitations. You tire easily. You get out of breath easily. This program is designed with you in mind. Most of the exercises are done seated in a chair. There are a few standing exercises, BUT if you find that you cannot do those, all you have to do is email me and I will walk you through those exercises while being seated. Most of the exercises can be done while being seated, standing or lying on the floor - depending on your specific physical limitations. You can catch Ellen on www.uanetwork.tv on Mondays at 10:30

FIT&FAB LIVING

Emilie Yount | Editor

emiliey@silvercarrot.com

http://www.FitandFabLiving.com

Fit&Fab Living

Our dedicated editorial team is devoted to helping you look and feel your best by providing you with trusted information on a variety of health and beauty topics. We believe that there are many parts to wellness including physical health, mental well-being and exuberant self-confidence. At Fit&Fab Living, you can access thousands of free beauty tips, health articles, delicious recipes and workout plans for all ages and levels to help you live each and every day feeling your absolute best! We seek out health professionals and fitness experts to obtain only the very best advice. Our blog Running with Mascara is a source of fashion and beauty advice, expert opinions and sweepstakes for everything from beauty products to healthy snacks.

After a long day of work, coming home to your favorite reality television show or medical drama can be a comforting way to spend the evening. It's easy to plan to workout in the evening and then let the rush of fatigue wash over you as you snuggle up to the couch for the next few hours. It's tough to decide between the comfort of watching your favorite shows and the workout you know you need. No need to choose anymore because Fit&Fab Living has come up with the perfect solution - workout while you watch TV!

Television Toners

A 30-minute television program has about 10 minutes of commercials! You can either workout throughout the duration of the television episode, or if you're just beginning, start slowly and only workout during commercial breaks. You can gradually increase the time as you feel more comfortable. You can get all the enjoyment out of your shows and still burn calories, too. It does mean that you have to commit to movement during TV time, but we promise you'll feel a lot better knowing you've got the best of both worlds. Try some of these TV workout exercises and you'll notice the difference in your strength, flexibility and muscle tone.

If you have a treadmill, this is the easiest way to get in a great cardio workout. Place the treadmill in a spot where you can still see the television or move a smaller television in front of the treadmill and start walking! While you don't need to be huffing and puffing, you should be walking at a fairly brisk pace. If you're looking for a challenge, raise the incline! If you don't have a treadmill, jog in place, do knee raises or jumping jacks. Do any or all of these exercises for 1 minutes intervals on and off until the show's over.

Pushups are a great muscle-building exercise. Try them on the floor for the greatest challenge or for a less strenuous option, do pushups standing up against a wall. Do as many as you can until your arms won't let you do one more!

Leg lifts are another easy option to tone thighs. Lie on your side with the bottom leg straight and the top leg slightly bent. Lift and lower leg 30 times on each side.

TV time is the perfect time to get in a killer ab workout. Try these abs exercises to start toning your abs.

If you're looking to sculpt your derriere, then do chair squats during commercial breaks. Stand up in front of a couch or chair and then squat down until you are almost sitting, but not quite. Stand back up and repeat for the length of the commercial break.

Pick up a set of dumbbells and you can really amp up your toning exercises by adding all kinds of arm-toning exercises to your routine.

{ *You can get all the enjoyment out of your shows and still burn calories, too.* }

SIT STRETCH SMILE

Dr. Howie Shareff

www.youcallthisyoga.org

919-522-2646

Email: Howie@youcallthisyoga.org

Sit Stretch Smile book and DVD provides any viewer with easy, chair yoga postures, breathing and movements to improve their life. This 64 page, easy to follow, full color book and 90 minute DVD of the book, allow people of limited or full mobility to live life more aligned and aware.

Chair Yoga Relieves Pain

Here is an interesting story. Practice this yourself, without pain, too. At a recent class, a new student arrived with moderate to severe pain in his neck and back. He suffered from a recent injury that resulted in pressure on the discs that support his spine. His movement was slow, his posture rigid, and he had limited ability to sit on a chair with comfort. The student was about 6'2" tall, in his 40's, good physical shape and familiar with breathing and martial arts. He had not practiced these disciplines recently nor was he familiar with yoga.

Following guidelines for chair yoga, I set him up on three stackable chairs to create the proper height of the seat relative to the length of his legs. This positioning reduced pressure on his lower back by having his knees just a bit lower than his thighs. Find a way for your feet to be flat on the floor and your hips a bit higher than your knees. Use a pillow or foot support. I placed a small rolled up towel in his lumbar area to re-establish the proper curve in his lower spine. This was touchy for him and took some adjustment to create the proper positioning without causing him to wince. Sitting Mountain Pose is essential for aligning the spine by positioning the hips under the spine and allowing the re-development of lumbar and cervical spine curves (they complement each other). Place a small rolled up towel behind your lower back. Play Lumbar Limbo by drawing your tail a bit under the towel as you inhale. Positioning the elbows under the shoulders and head over the shoulder area allows for less tension in the neck and upper back. Now the muscle that is often tense across the upper back can begin to relax.

We proceeded to develop a breathing practice where the exhales were slightly longer in length than the inhales. Inhale for a count of 4, pause a moment, exhale for a count of 6. Repeat. With permission, I guided his upper back muscles diagonally toward his spine and helped to settle the shoulder blades on to the back ribs with the exhale. The muscles were in such spasm that they spontaneously twitched. The breathing practice proceeded for several minutes. Eventually the tension in his face and whole body significantly diminished and the twitching ceased.

The next part of the practice was to develop gentle extension and flexion of the spine. This was accomplished with gentle Cat/Cow poses over several minutes and within his range of motion comfort zone. Once the hips were loose, we moved toward shoulder relaxation. The rolling the shoulders up from front to back and reversing this path, combined with a basic 6 pose flow, allowed for even more comfort. We finished the active phase by raising and lowering the shoulders while keeping the buns engaged during the exhale. He became taller, looser and relaxed.

We finished with a counting meditation to further calm his mind. By counting backward, one number at a time with each exhale, he was able to separate from the physical trauma and reduce pain.

{ *Eventually the tension in his face and whole body significantly diminished and the twitching ceased.* }

POWER PILATES

Email: adrianspowerpilates@gmail.com

www.adrianspowerpilates.com

twitter.com/adrianpilates

facebook.com/adrianspowerpilates

BUTT BRIDGE

-Lie on back

-Knees bent, bottom of feet on floor, arms to your sides (reaching away from your head)

-Slowly tucked your abs up and under your ribs, lifting the tailbone off the ground, followed by your lower back, and then ending with your mid back

-Slowly roll back down -- mid back, lower back, ending with tailbone (Note: Do not arch back)

• *TARGET AREAS: Legs, Butt, Abs, and Spine*

BYE BYE BUTT

-Sit up tall, engaging the abs (may be done lying down or standing)

-Swiftly contract/squeeze/pulse glutes

• *TARGET AREAS: Butt, Abs, Inner/Outer Thighs*

FLY FIERCE

-Lie flat on your stomach, extending legs all the way out and arms all the way forward (body is in one straight line)

-Slowly lift the arms and legs up, leaving lower chest and pelvis on the floor (no bends at arms and legs)

• *TARGET AREAS: Arms, Shoulders, Upper/Mid/Lower Back, Butt, Legs, Abs*

RAISING THE ROOF!

-Sit tall

- Engage abs (and transversus abdominis)

-Simply lift your arms up to the ceiling and back down to shoulder level. Fists remain pointing to ceiling. (note: if in a car, extend as high as you can)

- Optional: use light dumbbells for more of a challenge. If not, gravity is heavy enough!

•*TARGET AREAS: shoulders, abs, obliques, back, and butt*

SPREAD YOUR WINGS

- Sit tall

- Engage abs (and transversus abdominis)

- Simply lift your arms up to the ceiling and slowly extend, reaching long, to both sides. Keep elbows straight.

- Optional: use light dumbbells for more of a challenge. If not, gravity is heavy enough!

• *TARGET AREAS: shoulders, chest, abs, obliques, back, and butt*

TUG-OF-WAR
- Sit tall
- Engage abs (and transversus abdominis)
- Extend arms in opposite directions, keeping the body tall, long, and upright (note: if in a car, you will need to lower your window to achieve optimal length)
- Slowly move your arms in circles, without bending your elbows. Repeat going the opposite direction.
• *TARGET AREAS: shoulders, arms, abs, obliques, back, and butt*

TWIST AWAY
- Sit tall
- Engage abs (and transversus abdominis)
- Position arm in from of you, with fists at your face. Imagine you're a boxer trying to protect your face.
- Twist from side to side, creating height and space between each vertabrae
• *TARGET AREAS: abs and obliques*

CONCLUSION

When I faithfully asked the question, what kind of lazy exercises I can do, I would never had believed I would have received such an overwhelming response. Never in a million years would I have thought a book would materialize. Never would I have thought that we can all have customized programs just for us. Since embarking on this journey it has now evolved into a passion of mine to find health and wellness programs for the underserved markets.

Yes, I am the first to admit I am sedentary. I sit at a desk all day long. Yes, I will admit I hate exercising and rather do something more exciting but I realize I want to get fit and healthy and I have to move, everyday deliberately.

I am sure I am not the only person who needs to exercise in a different way and constantly looking for new tools to help. Folks, there are plans out there. Maybe not readily under our feet, or marketed on TV but they are out there.

In conclusion it has been a terrific ride but it simply does not stop at a book. This has to go further.

I know people who have arthritis, bad back problems, knee injuries, fibromyalgia, senior citizens, office workers and home base entrepreneurs. We exist. We want good quality programs and we want supplements that will enhance and change our lives for better without any added chemicals.

In conclusion it has been a terrific ride but it simply does not stop at a book. This has to go further. We would not have so many unfit people if they realize there are programs out there for them. The people in the health and fitness industry you are all on notice. We need for you to make an effort to market to those of us who want a fit and healthy life but tailored for our needs and capabilities.

> *We would not have so many unfit people if they realize there are programs out there for them.*

If you have products, services and programs for people with health issues, sedentary, senior citizens, office workers, home base entrepreneur, chronic pain sufferer or morbidly obese, we want to hear from you. Please email us at info@allaboutmefitness.com.

If you are one of the many people who want custom fitness, we like to hear from you as well. Please email us at info@allaboutmefitness.com.com. Tell us how your customize plans are working and drop us a line if you want access to more experts in the health and fitness field.

Thanks for purchasing this book. Do you know you fed an American and gave a toy to a child? When you purchased this book some of the proceeds went to Feeding America and Toys for Tots. For that I say, thank you!

Questions You Should Ask When Choosing Your Health and Fitness Expert

Outside your exercise program will you recommend an eating program?

If I decide to hire you as my fitness coach, can you tell me exactly what that entails?

Why are you recommending these supplements, live food or tools for me?

How often do you check on your clients once they are utilizing your services?

I have not exercised in years so what type of movements will be safe for me?

I see these supplements will give you energy, what exactly is in them?

Are they safe and natural?

Will they interfere with my medicines?

Do you periodically send tips/articles/videos geared just for me?

Have you studied or done research on my condition?

Sometimes with my condition I can have good days and bad, can you adapt your plans for how I am doing at the moment?

How long have you been creating programs for people with my condition?

Do you know some natural pain management techniques?

Are your exercise programs safe for someone like me?

Of the different types of movements are there one or more that you recommend I do and some you don't recommend?

Will this supplement change any of the composition of my medicines?

How do you test your products?

Do you have access to a medical doctor or physician assistant for information and techniques?

Is there a facility in my city that you can recommend for me for added support?

Can I talk to any of your clients, past or present?

Disclaimer

This book is intended as a reference volume only, not as a medical manual. The information given here is designed to help you make informed decisions about your health. It is not intended as a substitute for any treatment that may have been prescribed by your doctor.

Before starting any exercise program or before taking any supplements or using tools please check with your doctor first.

Mention of specific companies, organizations, or authorities in this book does not imply endorsements by the publisher, nor does mention of specific companies, organizations, or authorities in the book imply that they endorse the book. Mention of particular brands does not imply endorsements by the publisher.

It is always recommended that you seek advice from your doctor or health advisor before beginning any new supplement or exercise regimen.

If you are exercising from a chair please make sure the chair is stable and remain cautious at all times.

Internet addresses and telephone numbers given in the book were accurate at the time the book went to press.

About the Author

Denise L. Jackson is a Certified Life/Career Coach and a Certified Green Consultant. She has worked in the banking and finance industry for more than 15 years training interns and new graduates. She decided to

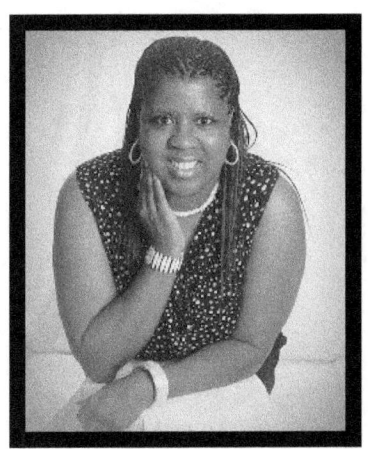

embark on a new career coaching teens and young adults and soon started Enhance My Skills, an e-mentoring/e-coaching online company preparing teens and young adults for the marketplace. Quickly afterwards she created Mo-Active Learning Series which is a series of workbooks that combines motivation, activation and skills building for teens and young adults.

Denise also has a heart for the environment and started offering high schools, workforce agencies, training centers and nonprofits Certified Entry Level Green Jobs Training. She is the author of Bringing Sexy to Green! We like to hear from you. Visit us at www.deniseljackson.com or www.enhancemyskills.com. Visit her blog at www.deniseljackson.wordpress.com. If you are a fitness expert who customizes exercise programs for the people mentioned in this book or if you have products, services and tools that can help a person maintain fitness and health, we like to hear from you. Please email us info@allaboutmefitness.com and put in subject line "Custom Fitness".